D1633238

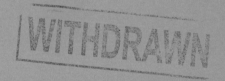

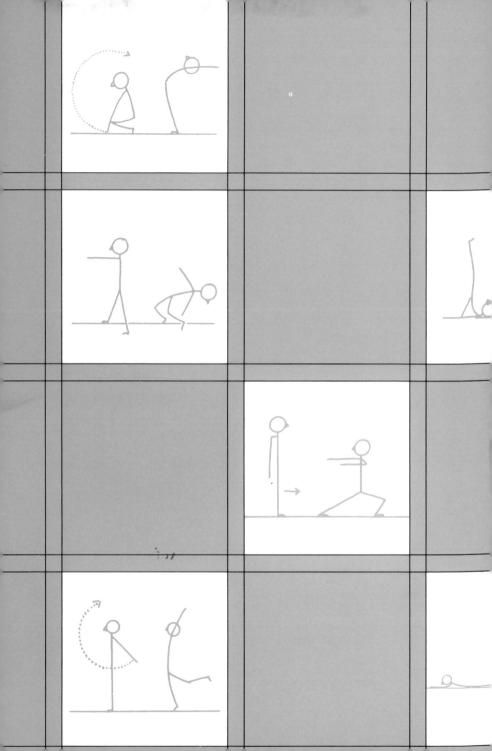

WARM-UP AND PREPARATION
FOR ATHLETES OF ALL SPORTS

*A Complete Book of Warm-up
and Flexibility Exercises*

By
Zoltan Tenke
Andy Higgins

Illustrations by
Eric Little

SPORT BOOKS PUBLISHER TORONTO

Canadian Cataloguing in Publication Data

Tenke, Zoltan
  Warm-up and preparation for athletes of all sports

ISBN 0-920905-44-7

1. Exercise.   I. Higgins, Andy.   II. Title

GV461.T45 1994   613.71   C94-930252-X

Distribution worldwide by
Sport Books Publisher
278 Robert Street
Toronto, Ontario M5S 2K8 Canada

Printed in the United States

CONTENTS

THE NEED FOR A WARM-UP

A warm-up routine prepares the athlete for more intense movements requiring speed and strength. It is designed to gradually adjust his/her organism to more effectively cope with relatively high physical demands. Therefore, an adequate warm-up is important for all athletic activities, whether it be a training session or a competition.

In any athletic activity it is important to gradually increase the intensity of effort, so that the gradually prepared organism is less susceptible to injury of muscles and related tissue, and capable of much higher levels of performance.

All activity necessitates an increased rate of fuel consumption in the organism, specifically in the muscles involved. This is above the normal metabolic processes at rest. An ongoing, increased rate of fuel consumption is only possible when the arteries deliver the nutritive material at a faster rate. This can only be achieved gradually by following a well designed warm-up routine. It is the easily begun, gradually increased activity during the warm-up that stimulates the nervous system and gives it time to set into action this delivery process. As the body temperature rises, the heart rate is increased, and the arteries and capillaries are opened with a resultant increase in the volume of blood flowing to the muscles and delivering nutritive material (oxygen and fuel foods) at a higher rate.This brings about an equal response in the nervous system to more quickly remove metabolic wastes from the muscles.

If the athlete does not gradually increase the intensity of work using a well designed warm-up routine, initially his/her circulatory system cannot possibly function in physiologically most efficient ways. This insufficient preparation of the circulatory system has a negative two-fold effect. Firstly, stored energy fuels must be consumed in the early stages of activity, and secondly, wastes are not removed quickly enough. Both these situations may contribute to a very early feeling of fatigue. This lack of a proper warm-up prior to vigorous activity creates a situation in which the athlete cannot perform maximally for the first few minutes, not until the system becomes adjusted to this new, higher level. It is not necessary to explain the disadvantages of this situation in competitive sports.

Another major consideration is the possibility of injuries to muscles and related tissue due to a lack of preparation. In a normal situation (i.e., sitting, standing, walking, etc.) the organism is in a relative state of rest. There is a degree of stiffness or tightness in the muscles and related connective tissues, and movements at the joints are somewhat restricted. This is also related to the generally lower level of circulation which exists in the muscles, making them and their related tissue much more susceptible to injury. Through warm-up activities, the blood supply at the specific tissue level is increased, and the muscle fibres become more relaxed and elongated, i.e., more prepared to withstand the demands of activity, more prepared to move easily and quickly.

In summary, a good warm-up prepares the athlete for higher levels of performance and lessens the likelihood of strains and tears to muscles and related tissue and sprains to the connective tissue at the joints.

PREPARATION

A warm-up routine has two phases, a general preparation phase, and a specific preparation phase.

1 General Preparation Phase

The main activities of the general preparation phase include walking, jogging, easy running, and calisthenics exercises.

The warm-up is begun with walking, jogging, and easy running because these activities serve as an excellent transition from rest to low level activity. These are good beginning movements since they quickly stimulate activity in the circulo-respiratory system (heart and lungs). With this heightened metabolism we are now ready to begin the calisthenics exercises which will further stimulate general circulation and prepare the muscles specifically and the systems generally for an even higher level of work. These calisthenics exercises are to be done with ease and reasonable effort, and are primarily designed to loosen and stretch the muscles and related tissue. Exercises for all major parts of the body should be completed; lower and upper limbs, and the trunk. For example, to warm-up the trunk necessitates the use of numerous different exercises that bend and rotate the body in all the different planes. Consequently, the whole body must be warmed up, all muscles and all joints regardless of the particular sport. For example, in hockey, which primarily involves skating and shooting, it is necessary to be prepared for that sudden, unexpected twisting of the trunk to avoid a check. It is the unprepared athlete who thus acquires minor muscle pulls in the lower back or trunk that can impede performance for days or even weeks.

This general preparation is essential no matter what the activity , although we recognize that many sports have additional, specific requirements that necessitate more attention be paid to particular body areas. On occasion, pick-up games, various contests, and relays may be used as part of the general warm-up with some calisthenics used to fulfill the requirements not already met.

The general warm-up may be concluded with a few accelerated runs.

2 Specific Preparation Phase

The activities of the specific preparation phase consist of exercises that closely simulate actions specific to a sport or event. After the general preparation, the athlete must then prepare both physically and mentally for the specific demands of his/her activity. Therefore, it is absolutely essential that the athlete does some exercises or drills that simulate parts of the specific activity, sport, or discipline, so as to activate the proper neuro-muscular mechanisms and, in a sense, test them and break them in, i.e., prepare them for the upcoming demands. For example, the football player may perform many passes or kicks, run short sprints, etc.; the basketball player may concentrate more on leaps and runs; the jumper does leaps and bounding exercises. In track and field, it is possible for all athletes to do the general preparation together, but they would have to break up into various event groups for the specific preparation.

In a training session, the specific preparation blends into the body of the workout. In a competitive situation, the specific preparation is the final effort immediately prior to the actual event.

HOW TO USE THIS BOOK

This book is concerned with calisthenics exercises related to the general warm-up. The general warm-up should always be based on the following coaching and physiological principles:

1. The different muscle groups and joints should be adequately warmed-up with a variety of exercises that take into consideration the total range of use. Each exercise is to be repeated about 8 -10 times to derive the proper effect. However, this is only a guide, as the athlete must feel that he/she has increased the range of movement(s) sufficiently. It takes about 10 - 15 minutes of calisthenics exercises to prepare adequately. It is important to keep in mind that the purpose of this activity is to prepare the organism, not to tire it out.

2. Each muscle group and joint area must be dealt with several times. Exercises for the upper limbs, trunk, and the lower limbs should be alternated; do not ignore any area for too long a time. If a muscle group is left out of the action for too long, the effectiveness of the warm-up is reduced. The repeated activity in each area must ensure that all of the possible movement directions are involved.

3. The warm-up should begin with easy stretching exercises. This is a good time to use complex exercises that will involve various parts of the body and therefore several muscle groups.

4. There should not be undue breaks between the exercises. Young athletes and unconditioned athletes need to take short breaks, but the highly conditioned athletes should remain active throughout the entire warm-up period.

5. The full benefit of these exercises can only be derived when they are performed correctly. The athlete will receive benefit from his/her warm-up in accordance with the thought and effort put into it. A lazily performed warm-up will produce minimal results.

6. Each individual exercise must begin gently and easily and increase in intensity and amplitude of motion only after the first few repetitions. For example, leg swinging will always start with easy swings, and only after a few swings will the leg be moved through as wide a range of motion as possible. This principle applies to the entire warm-up as well. It must begin gently and only increase in intensity as it progresses.

7. If there is more than 5 - 10 minutes between the completion of the warm-up and the beginning of the main activity, the athlete must do some further activity to avoid losing the benefits of the warm-up (i.e., jogging, hopping, skipping, arm-swinging, etc.).

8. Cold, windy and wet weather will necessitate more carefully planned and longer warm-up periods. These are the weather conditions which precipitate injuries and special precautions must be taken. It is important to perform the full warm-up and then maintain the preparation state right up to the beginning of more intense activity (workout or competition). During the warm-up, several 30 metre walks or jogs can be taken between exercises as an activity bridge.

9. When very hot weather is prevalent, fewer exercises need to be done, and the number of repetitions can be reduced to four or five.

10. The warm-up suit, so important on cold days, has value on warmer days as well, in maintaining a fairly consistent body temperature.

11. Considerations in developing a warm-up routine include the age, sex, general condition, and innate flexibility of the athlete. Generally, women and young children are more flexible than males, and require less specific flexibility exercises. The warm-up must be suited to the needs of the individual.

EXERCISE GROUPS

This manual has 15 sections dealing with the varying exercise effects and body areas. Each section deals specifically with one type of exercise (i.e., hopping), or one body area (i.e., shoulders), or one effect (i.e., strength). If one exercise is selected from each of the 15 groups, one can prepare all the major muscle groups around all the joint areas.

The major exercise groups presented are:

1. Hopping Exercises
2. Arm- Pulling Exercises
3. Trunk- Bending Exercises - Forwards
4. Leg- Swinging Exercises - Forwards
5. Trunk- Bending Exercises - Backwards
6. Arm- Swinging and Circling Exercises
7. Trunk- Twisting Exercises
8. Leg- Swinging Exercises - Backwards
9. Trunk- Bending Exercises - Laterally
10. Leg- Swinging Exercises - Laterally and Circling
11. Combination Exercises
12. Knee- Bouncing or Springing Exercises
13. Arm and Shoulder Girdle Strengthening Exercises
14. Abdominal and Lower Trunk Strengthening Exercises
15. Back and Lower Trunk Strengthening Exercises

Each group presents 12 sample exercises. They are generally exhibited in an order of increasing difficulty. The coach or instructor can select one exercise from each group, and prepare a 10 - 15 minute warm-up program. The possibilities for varying this warm-up routine are many.

Exercises in groups 1 to 12 will generate a complete warm-up. In hot weather conditions, it is wise to omit the complex exercises illustrated in group 11. Exercises in groups 13 to 15 are strengthening activities and should be used with caution and only in relation to the main activity of the day. For example, it would not be necessary or wise to engage in strengthening exercises immediately prior to competition.

As a general rule, it is wise to change the exercises in the general warm-up routine as often as necessary to prevent boredom, while continuing to meet the demands of the situation.

BODY POSITIONS AND STANCES

All the basic warm-up and preparation exercises described commence from one of seven body positions or stances. They are:

1. Basic Erect Stance
2. Basic Sitting Position
3. Basic Kneeling Position
4. Squat
5. Basic Prone Position
6. Basic Supine Position
7. Jogging, described as 'While Jogging'

Most of the basic positions or stances have variations wherein the limbs are placed in a specific position to facilitate the exercise. These variations are:

1. Straddle, i.e., legs apart;
2. Deep Straddle, i.e., similar to the straddle, but with legs further apart;
3. Support, i.e., arms placed on the ground to support the body;
4. Split, i.e., legs apart, but one in front of the other.

Examples of each of the basic body positions and stances are illustrated on pages 14 to 19.

1 Basic Positions

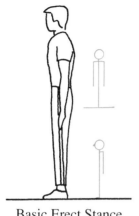

Basic Erect Stance

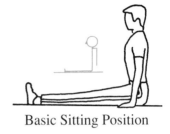

Basic Sitting Position

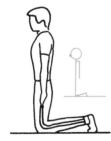
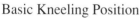

Basic Kneeling Position

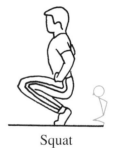

Squat

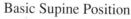

Basic Supine Position

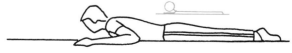

Basic Prone Position

2 Straddle Positions

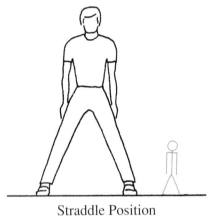

Straddle Position

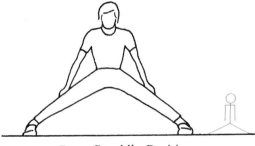

Deep Straddle Position

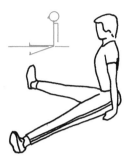

Sitting Straddle Position

Prone Straddle Position

Supine Straddle Position

3 Support Positions

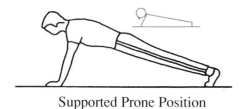

Supported Prone Position

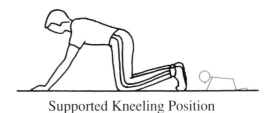

Supported Sitting Position

Supported Kneeling Position

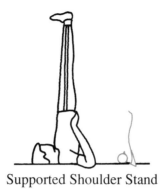

Supported Shoulder Stand

Supported Squat

ARM POSITIONS

All basic stances or positions, i.e., Basic Erect Stance, require the arms to be placed at the sides of the body. However, some of the exercises demand that the starting position of the arms be different. These are as follows:

1. High Position
2. Side Shoulder Position
3. Forward Position
4. Deep Diagonal Position
5. Crossed in Front of Body
6. Hands on Chest
7. High Diagonal Position
8. Low Diagonal Position
9. Deep Front Diagonal Position
10. Arms Akimbo
11. Hands on Shoulders
12. Hands Directly Beneath Shoulders

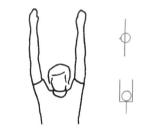

Arms in High Position

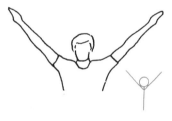

Arms in High Diagonal Position

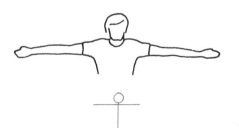
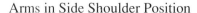

Arms in Side Shoulder Position

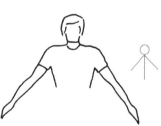

Arms in Low Diagonal Position

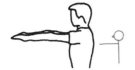

Arms in Forward Position

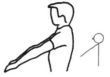

Arms in Deep Front
Diagonal Position

Arms in Deep
Diagonal Position

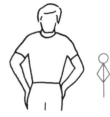

Arms Akimbo

Arms Crossed in
Front of Body

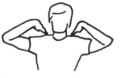

Hands on Shoulders

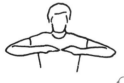

Hands on Chest

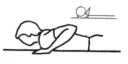

Hands Directly
Beneath Shoulders

EXERCISE POOL

1 Hopping Exercises

E1 From a Basic Erect Stance:
Hop twice with feet together on '1 -
2', and twice with feet straddled on
'3 - 4'. Done to a '1 -2 - 3 - 4' rhythm.

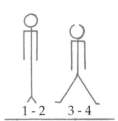

**E2 From a Split Stance, with left foot
forward:**
Hop twice with left foot forward on
'1 - 2', and twice with right foot forward on '3 - 4'. As in E1, done to a
'1 - 2 - 3 - 4' rhythm.

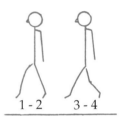

E3 From a Basic Erect Stance:
Hop 3 times with legs together on '1 -
2 - 3', and a high hop on '4'.

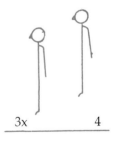

E4 From a Basic Erect Stance:
Hop 3 times with legs together on '1 -
2 - 3', and a high hop on '4' with
heels brought up to buttocks.

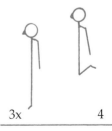

E5 **From a Basic Erect Stance:**
Hop 3 times with legs together on '1 -
2 - 3', and a high hop with arms in
side shoulder position and legs straddled on '4'. Land with feet together.

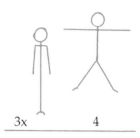

E6 **From a Basic Erect Stance:**
Hop 3 times with legs together on '1 -
2 - 3', and land in a deep, front supported squat position on '4'.

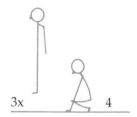

E7 **From a Basic Erect Stance:**
Hop twice on left foot keeping right
knee high on '1 - 2'. Repeat with right
foot on '3 - 4'.

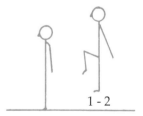

E8 **From a Basic Erect Stance:**
Hop twice on left foot, with right leg
swinging outwards, on '1 - 2'. Repeat
with right foot on '3 - 4'.

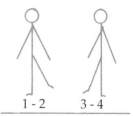

**E9   From an Erect Stance, with arms in
Side Shoulder Position:**
Hop with feet together and swing arms
down to a crossed pose in front of
trunk on '1'. Repeat hop, raising arms
to starting position on '2'.

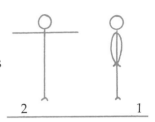

**E10 From an Erect Stance, with arms in
Deep Diagonal Position:**
Hop with feet together and swing arms
forwards to shoulder height on '1'.
Repeat hop, swinging arms to starting
position on '2'.

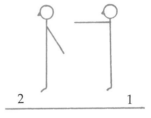

**E11 From an Erect Stance, with arms in
Deep Diagonal Position:**
Hop with legs together three times on
'1 - 2 - 3', and a high hop with complete
arm rotation forwards and back on '4'.

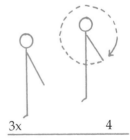

E12 From a Basic Erect Stance:
Hop 3 times with legs together on '1 -
2 - 3', and a high hop with knees
brought up to chest in clasped tuck
position on '4'.

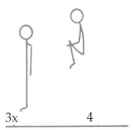

2 Arm-Pulling Exercises

**E1   From an Erect Stance, with Hands
on Shoulders:**
Arms bent, pull elbows to rear twice
on '1 - 2'. Pull arms straight to rear on
'3 - 4'. Done to a '1 - 2 - 3 - 4'
rhythm.

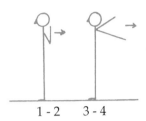

1 - 2   3 - 4

**E2   From an Erect Stance, with Hands
on Chest:**
Circle elbows backwards twice on
'1 - 2'. Pull arms straight to rear twice
on '3 -4'. As in E1, done to a
'1 - 2 - 3 - 4' rhythm.

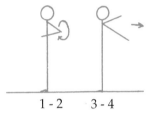

1 - 2   3 - 4

**E3   From an Erect Stance, with arms in
Side Shoulder Position:**
Pull straight arms to rear twice on
'1 - 2'. Clap hands behind back twice
on '3 - 4'.

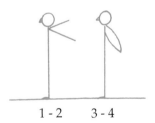

1 - 2   3 - 4

**E4   From an Erect Stance, with arms in
Side Shoulder Position:**
Swing arms across front of trunk on
'1'. Return to starting position on
'2'. Pull straight arms to rear twice on
'3 - 4'.

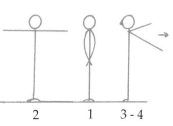

2   1   3 - 4

E5 From an Erect Stance, with arms in Side Shoulder Position:
Pull straight arms backwards twice on '1 - 2'. Swing arms above head and press backwards on '3 - 4'.

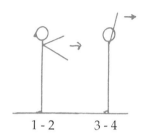

1 - 2   3 - 4

E6 From an Erect Stance, with one arm in High Position:
Press arms backwards twice on '1 - 2'. Change arm positions and repeat backwards arm presses twice on '3 - 4'.

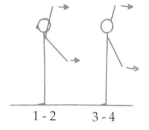

1 - 2   3 - 4

E7 From an Erect Stance, with arms in High Position:
Swing arms sideways and downwards to a crossed position in front of trunk on '1'. Return arms to high position on '2'. Press arms backwards twice on '3 - 4'.

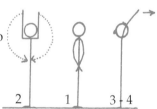

2   1   3 - 4

E8 From an Erect Stance, with arms in Deep Diagonal Position:
Swing arms forwards to a position above the head, pressing three times on '1 - 2 - 3'. Return to starting position and press arms backwards on '4'.

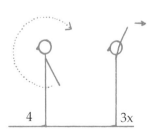

4   3x

**E9 From an Erect Stance, with arms in
Low Diagonal Position:**
Press arms backwards twice on '1 - 2'.
Raise arms to high diagonal position
and press backwards twice on '3 - 4'.

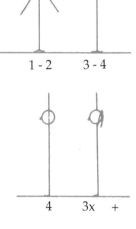

**E10 From an Erect Stance, with arms in
High Diagonal Position:** (See second
figure in E9.) Bend left elbow backwards so (left) hand touches left shoulder blade 3 times on '1 - 2 - 3'. Return
to starting position on '4'. Repeat exercise with right hand to touch right shoulder blade to a '1 - 2 - 3 - 4' rhythm.

**E11 From an Erect Stance, with arms in
Deep Diagonal Position:**
Swing arms to side, shoulder height, and
press backwards on '1'. Swing to high
position and press backwards on '2'.
Return to shoulder height position and
press backwards on '3'. Return to starting position and press backwards on '4'.

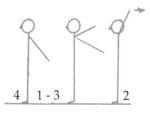

**E12 From an Erect Stance, with hands
behind back, fingers interlocked,
palms outwards:**
Press arms up and back three times on
'1 - 2 - 3'. Return to starting position
on '4'.

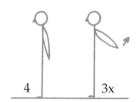

3 Trunk-Bending Exercises – Forwards

E1 **From an Erect Straddle Stance, with arms in Side Shoulder Position:**
Bend forwards to touch ankles 3 times on '1 - 2 - 3'. Return to starting position on '4'.

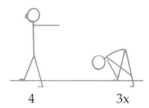

4   3x

E2 **From an Erect Straddle Stance, with arms in Side Shoulder Position:**
Bend forwards and reach left hand to ground between legs 3 times on '1 - 2 - 3'. Return to starting position on '4'. Repeat with right arm to a '1 - 2 - 3 - 4' rhythm.

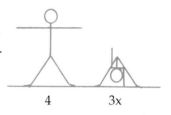

4   3x

E3 **From an Erect Straddle Stance, with arms in Side Shoulder Position:**
Bend forwards to touch both hands to ground between legs 3 times on '1 - 2 - 3'. Return to starting position on '4'.

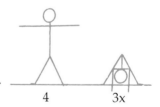

4   3x

E4 **From an Erect Straddle Stance, with arms in High Position:**
Swing forwards and press both arms backwards between legs 3 times on '1 - 2 - 3'. Return to starting position on '4'.

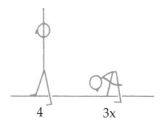

4   3x

**E5 From an Erect Straddle Stance,
with arms in High Position:**
Bend forwards to touch both hands to
left ankle 3 times on '1 - 2 - 3'. Return
to starting position on '4'. Repeat with
both hands to right ankle to a '1 - 2 - 3
- 4' rhythm.

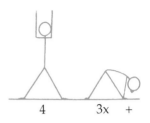

4   3x   +

**E6 From an Erect Stance, with arms in
High Position:**
Bend forwards to touch toes 3 times
on '1 - 2 - 3'. Return to starting position on '4'.

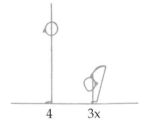

4   3x

**E7 From an Erect Straddle Stance, with
arms in Side Shoulder Position:**
Bend forwards to touch left hand to
right foot 3 times on '1 - 2 - 3'. Return
to starting position on '4'. Repeat right
hand to left foot. (Raised arm must
press backwards!)

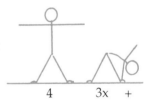

4   3x   +

**E8 From an Erect Straddle Stance,
with fingers interlocked behind
back, palms outwards:**
Bend forwards and press arms up and
backwards 3 times on '1 - 2 - 3'.
Return to starting position on '4'.

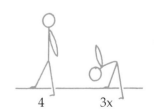

4   3x

E9 From a Supported Squat Position:
Raise hips to straighten knees and
touch toes 3 times on '1 - 2 - 3'.
Return to starting position on '4'.

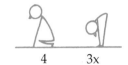

4   3x

**E10 From a Sitting Position, with arms
in High Position:**
Reach forwards to touch toes 3 times
on '1 - 2 - 3'. Return to starting position on '4'.

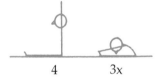

4   3x

**E11 From a Sitting Straddle Position,
with arms in Side Shoulder Position:**
Bend forwards with both arms touching left foot 3 times on '1 - 2 - 3'.
Return to starting position on '4'.
Repeat with both arms touching
right foot.

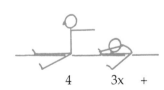

4   3x   +

**E12 From a Deep Straddle Stance, with
arms in Side Shoulder Position:**
Bend forwards to touch left elbow to
ground 3 times on '1 - 2 - 3'. Return
to starting position on '4'. Repeat with
right elbow.

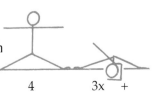

4   3x   +

4 Leg-Swinging Exercises – Forwards

E1 **From an Erect Stance, with arms in
Side Shoulder Position:**
Swing left leg forwards and up, clap-
ping hands together under leg on '1'.
Return to starting position on '2'.
Repeat with right leg on '3 - 4'.

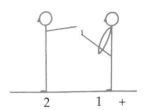

E2 **From an Erect Stance, with arms in
High Diagonal Position, palms
down:**
Swing left leg to touch left palm on
'1'. Return to starting position on '2'.
Repeat with right leg to right palm on
'3 - 4'.

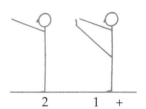

E3 **While jogging:**
Swing left leg forward and up on '1'.
Return to jogging on '2'. Repeat with
right leg on '3 - 4'.

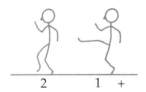

E4 **From an Erect Stance, with arms in
Side Shoulder Position:**
Swing both arms forwards and swing
left leg up to palms on '1'. Return to
starting position on '2'. Repeat with
right leg on '3 - 4'.

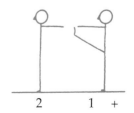

E5 **From a Supine Position, with knees bent and arms in High Diagonal Position:**
Swing left leg to touch left palm on '1'. Return to starting position on '2'. Repeat with right leg to right palm on '3 - 4'.

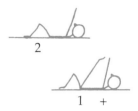

E6 **From a Supported Prone Position:**
Swing left leg sideways and forwards on '1'. Return to starting position on '2'. Repeat with right leg on '3 - 4'.

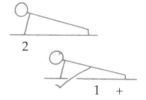

E7 **From a Supine Position, with arms in High Diagonal Position:**
Swing left leg to left palm on '1'. Return to starting position on '2'. Repeat with right leg to right palm on '3 - 4'.

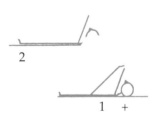

E8 **From a Prone Position, with arms in Side Shoulder Position, palms down:**
Swing left leg sideways and forwards to left hand on '1'. Return to starting position on '2'. Repeat with right leg to right hand on '3 - 4'.

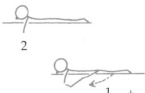

E9 From an Erect Stance, with arms in High Position:
Drop arms to horizontal position, and swing left leg to left palm on '1'. Return to starting position on '2'. Repeat with right leg to right palm on '3 - 4'.

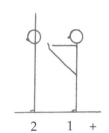

E10 From an Erect Stance, with arms in High Position:
Swing both arms down and backwards to a deep diagonal position as left leg swings up on '1'. Return to starting position on '2'. Repeat with arms but swing right leg on '3 - 4'.

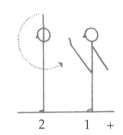

E11 From a Supine Position, with arms in Side Shoulder Position, palms down:
Swing left leg forwards and up, swing arms to grasp calf of leg, and pull leg to chest 3 times on '1 - 2 - 3'. Return to starting position on '4'. Repeat with right leg.

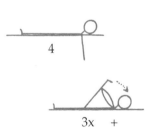

E12 While jogging:
Swing left leg forward and up to touch both hands as they swing forwards on '1'. Return to starting position on '2'. Repeat with right leg to touch hands on '3 - 4'. (Exercise requires trunk to bend slightly forwards.)

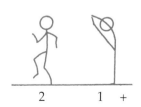

5 Trunk-Bending Exercises – Backwards

E1 From a Basic Straddle Stance:
Swing arms to side shoulder position,
palms down, and press trunk backwards 3 times on '1 - 2 - 3'. Return to
starting position on '4'.

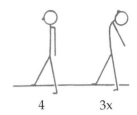

4   3x

**E2 From an Erect Straddle Stance,
with arms forwards:**
Swing arms to side shoulder position,
palms up, and press trunk backwards 3
times on '1 - 2 - 3'. Return to starting
position on '4'.

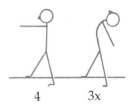

4   3x

E3 From a Basic Straddle Stance:
Swing left arm to high position and
press arm and trunk backwards 3
times on '1 - 2 - 3'. Return to starting
position on '4'. Repeat with right arm.

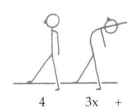

4   3x   +

E4 From a Basic Straddle Stance:
Placing bent right arm behind trunk,
swing left arm to high position, pressing arm and trunk backwards 3 times
on '1 - 2 - 3'. Return to starting position on '4'. Repeat with right arm,
placing bent left arm behind trunk.

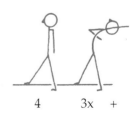

4   3x   +

E5 From a Basic Erect Stance:
Sidestep with left leg to straddle position, swing arms up to side shoulder position, palms up, and press trunk backwards 3 times on '1 - 2 - 3'.
Return to starting position on '4'.
Repeat with right leg.

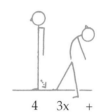

4   3x   +

E6 From a Kneeling Position, with knees slightly apart:
Swing arms to side shoulder position, palms up, and press trunk backwards twice on '1 - 2'. Bring trunk forwards on '3'. Return arms to side on '4'.

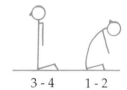

3 - 4   1 - 2

E7 From an Erect Straddle Stance, with arms in High Position:
Swing arms to side shoulder position with palms up, and press trunk backwards 3 times on '1 - 2 - 3'. Return to starting position on '4'.

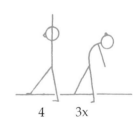

4   3x

E8 From an Erect Straddle Stance, with arms in Side Shoulder Position:
Swing arms to high position and press trunk backwards 3 times on '1 - 2 - 3'.
Return to starting position on '4'.

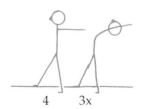

4   3x

E9 **From an Erect Stance, with arms in Deep Diagonal Position:**
Swing arms forwards, up and backwards, pressing trunk backwards 3 times on '1 - 2 - 3'. Return to starting position on '4'.

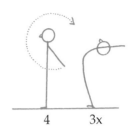

4   3x

E10 **From a Supported Squat Position:**
Extend knees, swing arms forwards, up and backwards, pressing trunk backwards 3 times on '1 - 2 - 3'. Return to starting position on '4'.

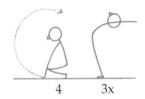

4   3x

E11 **From a Basic Straddle Stance:**
Swing arms up and backwards as trunk turns sideways, then presses backwards 3 times on '1 - 2 - 3'. Return to starting position on '4'.

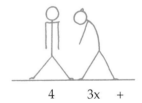

4   3x   +

E12 **From a Basic Straddle Stance:**
Bend knees, swing arms to side shoulder position, palms up, then press trunk backwards 3 times on '1 - 2 - 3'. Return to starting position on '4'.

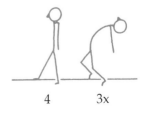

4   3x

6 Arm-Swinging and Circling Exercises

E1 **From an Erect Stance, with left arm in High Position:**
Swing arms backwards in windmill fashion, varying speed from slow to fast. (This exercise can also be done while walking or running on the spot.)

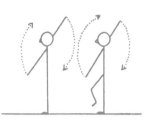

E2 **From an Erect Stance, with left arm in High Position:**
Swing arms forwards in windmill fashion, varying speed from slow to fast. (As in E1 above, this exercise can also be done while walking or running on the spot.)

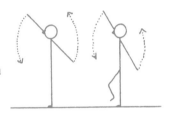

E3 **From an Erect Stance, with arms in Deep Diagonal Position:**
Swing both arms forwards on '1'. Swing arms in horizontal plane to side shoulder position on '2'. Swing arms to forward position on '3'. Return to starting position on '4'.

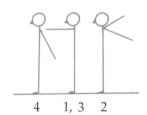

4   1, 3   2

E4 **From an Erect Stance, with arms in Deep Diagonal Position:**
Swing arms forwards on '1'. Return to starting position on '2'. Swing arms to high position and rise up on toes on '3'. Return to starting position on '4'.

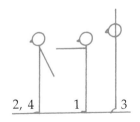

2, 4   1   3

E5 **From an Erect Stance, with arms in Side Shoulder Position:**
Drop arms to crossed position in front of trunk on '1'. Swing arms to side shoulder position on '2'. Swing arms forwards and down through two complete inward circles on '3 - 4'.

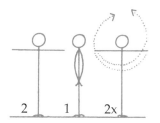

E6 **From an Erect Stance, with left arm in High Position:**
Swing arms forwards, thereby exchanging arm positions, varying speed from slow to fast.

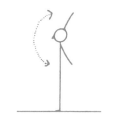

E7 **From an Erect Stance, with arms in Side Shoulder Position:**
Swing arms through a 1 1/2 inward circle to a crossed position in front of trunk on '1 - 2'. Return to starting position by swinging arms through a 1 1/2 outward circle on '3 - 4'.

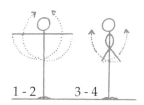

E8 **From an Erect Stance, with arms in High Position:**
Swing arms down and backwards to a deep diagonal position on '1'. Swing arms forwards, up and backwards to complete a circle on '2 - 3'. Continue circle to starting position on '4'.

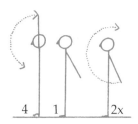

E9   From an Erect Stance, with arms in High Position:
Swing arms forwards through two circles on '1 - 2'. Swing arms backwards through two circles on '3 - 4'.

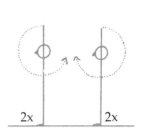

E10   From an Erect Stance, with arms in High Position:
Swing both arms down and across the body to the right twice on '1 - 2'. Swing both arms down and across the body to the left twice on '3 - 4'.

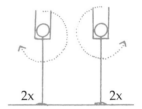

E11   From an Erect Straddle Stance, with arms in High Position:
Swing both arms down and across left side of body completing a circle on '1'. Swing both arms down and across right side of body completing a circle on '2'. Repeat the above on '3 - 4'. (This is a figure 8 motion.)

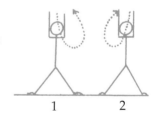

E12   From an Erect Straddle Stance, with arms in High Position:
Swing both arms outwards and down, completing a circle on '1 - 2'. Return to starting position, swinging arms in opposite circular fashion on '3 - 4'.

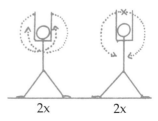

7 Trunk-Twisting Exercises

E1 From a Basic Straddle Stance:
Swing both arms to left side at shoulder height, and twist trunk with arms 3 times on '1 - 2 - 3'. Return to starting position on '4'. Repeat, swinging arms to right side.

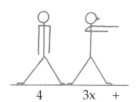

4   3x   +

E2 From a Basic Straddle Stance:
Clench right hand in front of chest, and clench left hand behind back, twisting to left side twice on '1 - 2'. Exchange arm positions and twist trunk twice to right side on '3 - 4'.

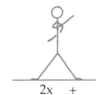

2x   +

E3 From an Erect Straddle Stance, with arms in High Position:
Drop left arm to side shoulder position, and rotate trunk to left side 3 times on '1 - 2 - 3'. Return to starting position on '4'. Repeat, rotating trunk to right side

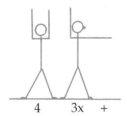

4   3x   +

E4 From an Erect Straddle Stance, with left arm in Side Shoulder Position, and right arm across chest:
Swing arms across body to right side, and twist trunk to the right 4 times on '1 - 2 - 3 - 4'. Bending forwards, repeat motion 4 times on '5 - 6 - 7 - 8' in vertical plane.

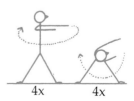

4x   4x

E5   From an Erect Straddle Stance, with arms in High Position:
Drop right arm across chest, drive arm and rotate trunk to left side 3 times on '1 - 2 - 3'. Return to starting position on '4'. Repeat, dropping left arm across chest, and driving arm and rotating trunk to right side.

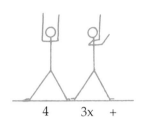

4   3x   +

E6   From a Kneeling Position, with knees apart, and arms in Forward Position:
Rotate trunk to left side, with left hand touching right ankle 3 times on '1 - 2 - 3'. Return to starting position on '4'. Repeat to right side.

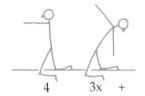

4   3x   +

E7   From a Supported Kneeling Position, with arms and thighs vertical to one another:
Swing left arm in side vertical plane above shoulder 3 times on '1 - 2 - 3'. Return to starting position on '4'. Repeat to right side.

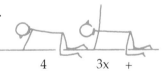

4   3x   +

E8   From a Straddle Stance, with arms in Forward Position:
Swing left arm and rotate trunk to left side, touching right ankle 3 times on '1 - 2 - 3'. Return to starting position on '4'. Repeat to right side.

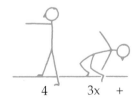

4   3x   +

E9   From a Deep Straddle Stance, with trunk bent forwards, palms on ground: Swing left arm and rotate trunk to left side 3 times on '1 - 2 - 3', while right palm remains on ground. Return to starting position on '4'. Repeat to right side.

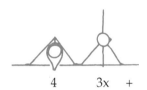

4   3x   +

E10 From a Sitting Straddle Position: Swing both arms to left side at shoulder height, and twist trunk with arms twice on '1 - 2'. Repeat to right side twice on '3 - 4'.

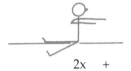

2x   +

E11 From a Basic Erect Stance: Take a long step forward with right foot, and swing both arms, rotating trunk to left side 3 times on '1 - 2 - 3'. Return to starting position on '4'. Repeat to right side, stepping forward with left foot.

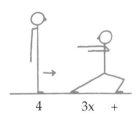

4   3x   +

E12 From a Prone Straddle Position, with arms in Side Shoulder Position, palms down: Swing left arm and rotate trunk to left side 3 times on '1 - 2 - 3'. Return to starting position on '4'. Repeat to right side.

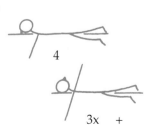

4

3x   +

8 Leg-Swinging Exercises –
Backwards

E1 While jogging:
Swing left leg backwards on '1'.
Return to jogging on '2'. Repeat,
swinging right leg backwards and
returning to jogging on '3 - 4'.

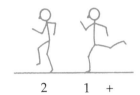

E2 From a Basic Erect Stance
Swing arms to side shoulder position,
and swing left leg backwards on '1'.
Return to starting position on '2'.
Repeat, swinging right leg backwards
and returning to starting position
on '3 - 4'.

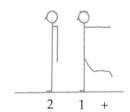

**E3 From an Erect Stance, with arms in
Deep Diagonal Position:**
Swing arms forwards to high position,
and left leg backwards on '1'. Return
to starting position on '2'. Repeat,
swinging right leg backwards and
returning to starting position on '3 -
4'.

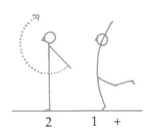

E4 From a Supported Squat Position:
Extend knees and raise hips, swinging
arms to side shoulder position and left
leg backwards on '1'. Return to starting position on '2'. Repeat, swinging
right leg backwards on '3 - 4'.

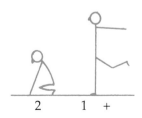

**E5 From a Supported Squat Position :
tion, with arms and thighs vertical
to one another:**
Swing left leg backwards to extended
position on '1'. Return to starting
position on '2'. Repeat, swinging right
leg backwards to extended position on
'3 - 4'.

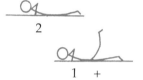

**E6 From a Basic Prone Position, with
hands directly beneath shoulders:**
Swing left leg backwards on '1'.
Return to starting position on '2'.
Repeat, swinging right leg backwards
on '3 - 4'.

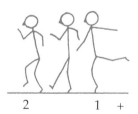

E7 While jogging:
Swing left leg slightly forwards and
from this position, swing leg backwards on '1'. Return to jogging on '2'.
Repeat with right leg on '3 - 4'.

E8 From Supported Squat Position:
Extend knees and raise hips, swinging
arms forwards to high position and left
leg backwards on '1'. Return to starting position on '2'. Repeat, swinging
right leg backwards on '3 - 4'.

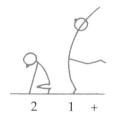

E9 **From a Basic Prone Position, with hands directly beneath shoulders:**
Swing left leg backwards on '1'.
Return to starting position on '2'.
Repeat swinging right leg backwards
on '3 - 4'.

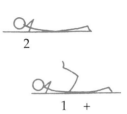

E10 **From a Supported Kneeling Position, with arms and thighs vertical to one another:**
Swing left leg backwards on '1'.
Swing left leg sideways and forwards
on '2'. Swing left leg backwards on
'3'. Return to starting position on '4'.
Repeat with right leg.

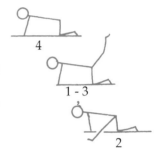

E11 **From an Erect Stance, with arms in Deep Diagonal Position:**
Swing arms forwards and sideways,
bending trunk backwards as left leg
swings backwards on '1'. Return to
starting position on '2'. Repeat with
right leg on '3 - 4'.

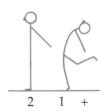

E12 **From a Supported Shoulder Stand:**
Swing left leg backwards 3 times on
'1 - 2 - 3'. Return to starting position
on '4'. Repeat with right leg.

9 Trunk-Bending Exercises – Laterally

E1   From a Basic Straddle Stance:
With right arm (elbow bent) swinging
laterally overhead, bend trunk to left
side 3 times on '1 - 2 - 3'. Return to
starting position on '4'. Repeat to
right side, with left arm (elbow bent)
swinging laterally.

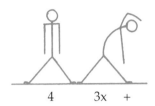

4   3x   +

**E2   From an Erect Straddle Stance,
with arms in High Position:**
Drop left arm to left knee, and bend
trunk to left side 3 times on '1 -2 - 3'.
Return to starting position on '4'.
Repeat, dropping right arm to right
knee, and bending trunk to right side.

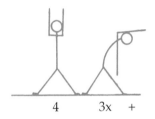

4   3x   +

E3   From a Basic Straddle Stance:
With left arm behind back and hand
clenched, swing bent right arm laterally overhead, bending trunk to left
side 3 times on '1 - 2 - 3'. Return to
starting position on '4'. Repeat, bending trunk to right side.

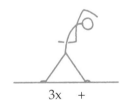

3x   +

**E4   From an Erect Straddle Stance, fin-
gers clasped on top of head:**
Extend arms and turn palms up as
trunk is bent to left side 3 times on '1 -
2 - 3'. Return to starting position on
'4'. Repeat, bending trunk to right
side.

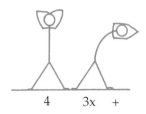

4   3x   +

E5   From a Basic Erect Stance:
Swing right arm laterally to high position, and bend trunk to left side 3
times on '1 - 2 - 3'. Return to starting
position on '4'. Repeat, bending trunk
to right side.

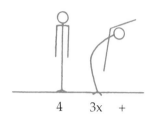

4   3x   +

**E6   From a Kneeling Position, with
arms in Side Shoulder Position:**
Bend trunk to left side, touching left
hand to floor 3 times on '1 - 2 - 3'.
Return to starting position on '4'.
Repeat, bending trunk to right side.

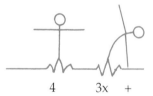

4   3x   +

**E7   From an Erect Stance, with arms in
High Position:**
Circle both arms to left side in front of
body twice on '1 - 2'. Bend trunk to
left side twice on '3 - 4'. Return to
starting position and repeat to right
side.

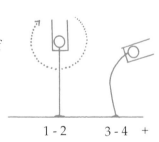

1 - 2   3 - 4   +

**E8   From an Erect Straddle Stance,
with arms Akimbo:**
Swing right arm laterally overhead,
bend right knee, and bend trunk to left
side 3 times on '1 - 2 - 3'. Return to
starting position on '4'. Repeat to
right side.

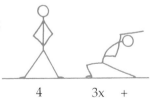

4   3x   +

**E9 From a Kneeling Position, with
arms in Side Shoulder Position:**
Extend left leg sideways, swing right
arm laterally overhead, and bend trunk
to left side 3 times on '1 - 2 - 3'.
Return to starting position on '4'.
Repeat to right side.

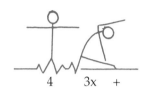

4   3x   +

E10 From a Supported Prone Position:
Bend left arm to hip, and drop right
hip 3 times on '1 - 2 - 3'. Return to
starting position on '4'. Repeat, bending right arm to hip, and dropping left
hip.

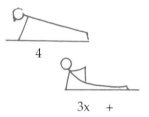

4

3x   +

E11 From a Basic Erect Stance:
With a lunge to right side, swing right
arm laterally overhead to bend trunk to
left side 3 times on '1 - 2 - 3', while
bending right knee. Return to starting
position on '4'. Repeat to right side.

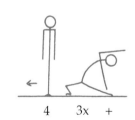

4   3x   +

E12 From a Basic Straddle Stance:
Swing right arm laterally overhead
and bend trunk to left side 3 times on
'1 - 2 - 3', bending left knee. Return to
starting position on '4'. Repeat to
right side.

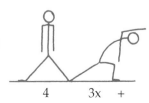

4   3x   +

10 Leg-Swinging Exercises – Laterally and Circling

E1   From an Erect Stance, with arms crossed in front of body:
Swing arms to side shoulder position, and swing left leg laterally on '1'. Return to starting position on '2'. Repeat with right leg on '3 - 4'.

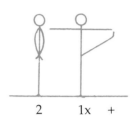

E2   From an Erect Straddle Stance, with arms in Side Shoulder Position:
Swing left leg across body to touch right hand on '1'. Return to starting position on '2'. Repeat with right leg on '3 - 4'.

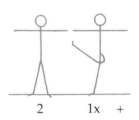

E3   From a Basic Prone Position, with hands directly beneath shoulders:
Swing left leg sideways and forwards to touch left hand on '1'. Return to starting position on '2'. Repeat with right leg on '3 - 4'.

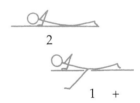

E4   From a Supine Position, with arms in Side Shoulder Position, palms down:
Swing left leg sideways to touch left hand on '1'. Return to starting position on '2'. Repeat with right leg on '3 - 4'.

**E5 From an Erect Stance, with arms
in Side Shoulder Position:**
Circle left leg forwards and outwards
on '1'. Return to starting position on
'2'. Repeat with right leg on '3 - 4'.

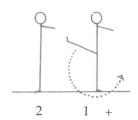

**E6 From a Supine Straddle Position,
with arms in Side Shoulder Position:**
Swing left leg to touch right hand on
'1'. Return to starting position on '2'.
Repeat with right leg to touch left
hand on '3 - 4'.

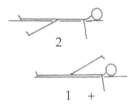

E7 From a Supported Squat Position:
Raise hips and swing arms to high
diagonal position while swinging left
leg laterally to diagonal position on
'1'. Return to starting position on '2'.
Repeat with right leg on '3 - 4'.

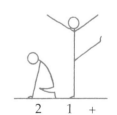

**E8 From a Prone Straddle Position,
with arms in Side Shoulder Position,
palms down:**
Swing right leg across back of left leg
to touch ground on '1'. Return to starting position on '2'. Repeat with left
leg touching ground on '3 - 4'.

E9 From an Erect Stance, with arms in Side Shoulder Position:
Circle left leg backwards and outwards on '1'. Return to starting position on '2'. Repeat with right leg on '3 - 4'.

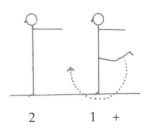

2   1   +

E10 From a Supported Prone Straddle Position:
Swing right leg across back of left leg to touch ground on '1'. Return to starting position on '2'. Repeat with left leg touching ground on '3 - 4'.

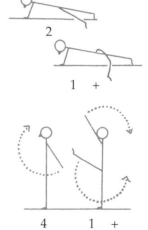

E11 From an Erect Stance, with arms in Deep Diagonal Position:
Circle arms forwards while circling left leg forwards on '1'. Circle arms overhead while circling left leg backwards twice on '2 - 3'. Return to starting position on '4'. Repeat with right leg.

4   1   +

E12 From a Basic Erect Stance:
Swing right arm laterally to high position, and bend trunk to left side as left leg swings laterally to left side on '1'. Return to starting position on '2'. Repeat to right side on '3 - 4'.

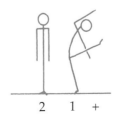

2   1   +

11 Combination Exercises

E1 **From a Basic Straddle Stance:**
Bend trunk forwards and touch ground
with both hands on '1 - 2'. Return to
starting position and swing both arms
to left and rotate trunk on '3 - 4'.
Repeat to right side.

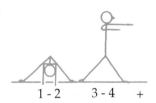

1 - 2   3 - 4   +

E2 **From a Basic Straddle Stance:**
Bend trunk forwards and touch ground
with both hands on '1 - 2'. Return to
starting position and swing right arm
laterally to overhead position, while
bending trunk to left side on '3 - 4'.
Repeat to right side.

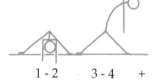

1 - 2   3 - 4   +

E3 **From an Erect Stance, with arms in
High Position:**
Swing both arms forwards, completing 3/4 circle and finish in deep diagonal position as trunk bends forwards
with knees bent on '1'. Return to starting position on '2'. Bend trunk backwards twice on '3 - 4'.

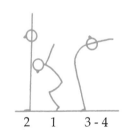

2   1   3 - 4

E4 **From an Erect Straddle Stance, with
arms in Side Shoulder Position:**
Maintaining a flat back, press trunk
forwards and down, keeping head up
and arms wide, on '1 - 2'. Bend trunk
to left side, touching left ankle with
both hands on '3 - 4'. Return to starting position and repeat to right side.

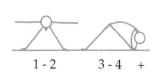

1 - 2   3 - 4   +

E5   From a Basic Straddle Stance:
With trunk bending to left side, touch
left ankle with both hands twice on
'1 - 2'. Rotating trunk to right side,
bend backwards twice with palms up
on '3 - 4'. Return to starting position
and repeat to right side.

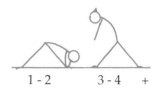

1 - 2   3 - 4   +

E6   From a Basic Straddle Stance:
Bending forwards, circle trunk to left
in counterclockwise direction on '1 - 2
- 3 - 4'. Repeat, circling trunk to right
in a clockwise direction.

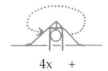

4x   +

E7   From a Basic Straddle Stance:
With trunk bending to left side, touch
left ankle with both hands twice on
'1 - 2'. Rotate trunk in a clockwise
direction on '3 - 4'. Repeat to right
side, rotating trunk counterclockwise.

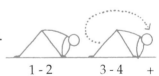

1 - 2   3 - 4   +

**E8   From a Supported Prone Straddle
Position:**
Rotate hips to the left in a circling
motion on '1 - 2 - 3 - 4'. Repeat to
right side.

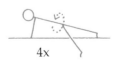

4x

E9   From a Basic Straddle Stance:
With trunk bending to left side, hold
left ankle with both hands. From this
position, swing *right arm* sideways,
turning trunk 3 times on '1 - 2 - 3'.
Return to starting position on '4'.
Repeat, from opposite starting position.

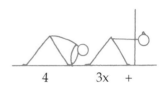

4   3x   +

E10 From a Basic Straddle Stance:
With trunk bending to left side, hold
left ankle with both hands. From this
position, swing *left arm* sideways,
turning trunk 3 times on '1 - 2 - 3'.
Return to starting position on '4'.
Repeat, from opposite starting position.

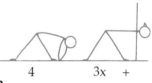

4   3x   +

**E11 From an Erect Straddle Stance, with
arms in Side Shoulder Position:**
Jump, and land in supported squat
position on '1'. Thrust legs backwards
into a supported prone straddle position on '2'. Return to supported squat
position on '3'. Jump to starting position on '4'.

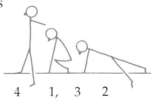

4   1, 3   2

E12 From a Basic Erect Stance:
Bend trunk forward, circling trunk
clockwise to left on '1 - 2 - 3 - 4'.
Repeat, circling trunk counterclockwise to right.

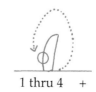

1 thru 4   +

12 Knee-Bouncing or Springing Exercises

E1 From an Erect Stance, with arms in Side Shoulder Position:
Lower trunk to a supported squat position, and execute 3 knee bounces on '1 - 2 - 3'. Return to starting position on '4'.

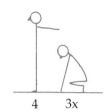

4   3x

E2 From an Erect Straddle Stance, with arms in Side Shoulder Position:
Jump to a supported squat position, and execute 3 knee bounces on '1 - 2 - 3'. Return to starting position on '4'.

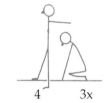

4   3x

E3 From an Erect Stance, with arms in High Position:
Lower trunk to a supported squat position, with left leg fully extended to the rear, and execute 3 knee bounces on right knee on '1 - 2 - 3'. Return to starting position on '4'. Repeat, extending right leg to rear.

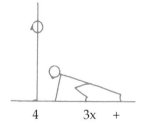

4   3x   +

E4 From an Erect Stance, with arms in High Position:
Jump to a supported squat position, and execute 3 knee bounces on '1 - 2 - 3'. Return with jump to starting position on '4'.

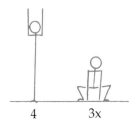

4   3x

E5 From a Basic Erect Stance:
Lunge to left side, and execute 3 knee
bounces on '1 - 2 - 3', touching
ground with both hands. Return to
starting position on '4'. Repeat to
right side.

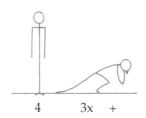

4   3x   +

E6 From a Basic Erect Stance:
Swing arms to side shoulder position,
lunge forwards with left leg and
bounce 3 times on '1 - 2 - 3'. Return
to starting position on '4'. Repeat with
right leg.

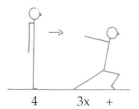

4   3x   +

E7 From a Supported Squat Position:
Execute 3 knee bounces on '1 - 2 - 3'.
Jump high with arms swinging for-
wards and up to high position on '4'.

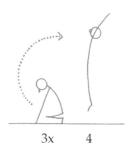

3x   4

E8 From a Supported Squat Position:
Extend left leg to rear and execute 2
knee bounces on right knee on '1 - 2'.
Exchange legs and execute 2 knee
bounces on left knee on '3 - 4'.

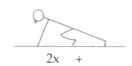

2x   +

E9   While jogging:
Lunge to left side and execute left
knee bounce, touching ground with
both hands 3 times on '1 - 2 - 3'.
Return to jogging position on '4'.
Repeat with lunge to right side.

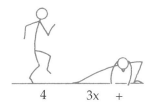

4   3x   +

E10 From a Supported Squat Position:
Execute 2 knee bounces on '1 - 2'.
Lunge forwards with left leg to supported position and execute 2 left knee
bounces on '3 - 4'. Repeat lunge with
right leg.

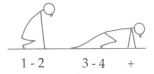

1 - 2   3 - 4   +

E11 From a Supported Squat Position:
Execute 2 bounces on '1 - 2'. Swing
arms to side shoulder position, lunge
to left side, and execute 2 left knee
bounces on '3 - 4'. Repeat lunge to
right side.

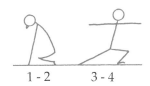

1 - 2   3 - 4

**E12 From a Squat Stance, with arms in
Side Shoulder Position:**
In this position, hop forwards on both
feet 4 times on '1 - 2 - 3 - 4'. Repeat,
hopping backwards on both feet 4
times in this position on '1 - 2 - 3 - 4'.

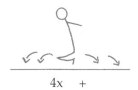

4x   +

13 Arm and Shoulder Girdle Strengthening Exercises

E1 **From a Supported Prone Position:**
Lower trunk on '1'. Return to starting
position on '2'. (This is a basic push-
up exercise.)

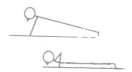

E2 **From a Supported Prone Straddle
Position:**
Lower trunk to touch forehead to
ground on '1 - 2'. Return to starting
position on '3 - 4'.

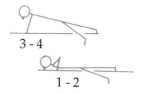

E3 **From a Supported Prone Straddle
Position:**
Reach forwards to touch ground with
left hand in front of shoulder 3 times
on '1 - 2 - 3'. Return to starting position on '4'. Repeat with right hand.

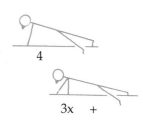

E4 **From a Supported Prone Straddle
Position:**
Reach sideways to touch ground with
left hand 3 times on '1 - 2 - 3'. Return
to starting position on '4'. Repeat with
right hand.

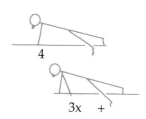

E5 From a Supported Prone Position:
Lower trunk as left leg is bent backwards on '1 - 2'. Return to starting
position on '3 - 4'. Repeat, bending
right leg backwards.

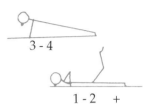

**E6 From a Supported Prone Straddle
Position:**
Drive vertically off the ground to clap
hands beneath chest on '1'. Return to
starting position on '2'. Repeat exercise on '3 - 4'.

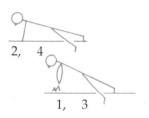

E7 From a Supported Prone Position:
Using the hands, walk a complete
circle to the left, around the legs.
Repeat to the right.

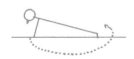

E8 From a Supported Prone Position:
Using the feet, walk a complete circle
to the left, around the hands. Repeat to
the right.

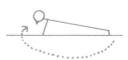

**E9   From a Supported Prone Straddle
Position, but using right arm only:**
Using the feet, walk a complete circle
to the left, around the right hand.
Exchange arms, and walk a complete
circle to the right, around the left
hand.

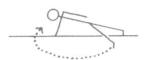

E10 From a Supported Squat Position:
Lower arms and extend legs to
achieve a basic prone straddle position
on '1'. Return, with jump, to starting
position on '2'. Repeat exercise on
'3 - 4'.

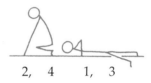

2,   4   1,   3

**E11 From a Supported Prone Straddle
Position:**
Drive vertically off the ground to clap
hands beneath chest, and to 'clap' feet
together on '1'. Return to starting
position on '2'. Repeat exercise on
'3 - 4'.

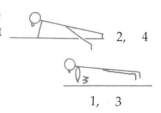

2,   4

1,   3

**E12 From a Deep Prone Straddle
Position, palms pressing ground:**
Push up trunk to a supported straddle
prone position on hands and toes on
'1'. Lower to starting position on '2'.
(This is an extended push-up.)

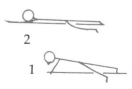

2

1

14 Abdominal and Lower Trunk Strengthening Exercises

E1 **From a Supported Sitting Position:**
Lift knees to touch forehead on '1'.
Extend legs to high diagonal position
on '2'. Lower legs to starting position
on '3 - 4'.

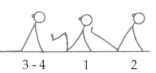

E2 **From a Basic Supine Position,
palms down:**
Lift both legs to vertical position on
'1 - 2'. Lower legs to starting position
on '3 - 4'.

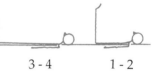

E3 **From a Basic Sitting Position, with
hands on hips:**
Lower trunk to a basic supine position
on '1 - 2'. Return to starting position
on '3 - 4'.

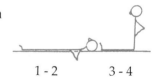

E4 **From a Supine Position, with arms
in High Position, palms up:**
Sit up, pull knees to chest, and clasp
hands in front of knees on '1 - 2'.
Return to starting position on '3 - 4'.

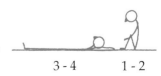

E5 **From a Supine Position, with arms in Side Shoulder Position, palms down:**
Sit up, lifting left knee to forehead on '1 - 2'. Return to starting position on '3 - 4'. Repeat, lifting right knee to forehead.

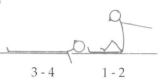

3 - 4   1 - 2

E6 **From a Basic Supine Position, palms down:**
Raise both legs to 30 degrees from horizontal position, scissoring legs with slow and fast rhythms.

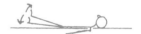

E7 **From a Supine Position, with arms in High Position, palms down:**
Sit up, bending trunk forwards to touch ankles on '1 - 2'. Return to starting position on '3 - 4'.

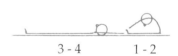

3 - 4   1 - 2

E8 **From a Supine Position, with arms in Deep Front Diagonal Position:**
Lift legs to 30 degrees from horizontal on '1'. Return to starting position on '2'. Lift trunk to 30 degrees from horizontal on '3'. Return to starting position on '4'.

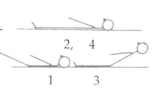

2, 4

1   3

E9   From a Basic Supine Position, palms down:
Raise both legs to touch ground over and behind head on '1 - 2'. Return to starting position on '3 - 4'.

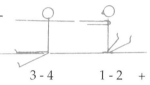

3 - 4   1 - 2

E10   From a Sitting Straddled Position, with arms in Side Shoulder Position:
Raise both legs and swing to left side as both arms swing to right side on '1 - 2'. Return to starting position on '3 - 4'. Repeat to opposite side.

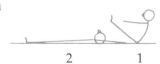

3 - 4   1 - 2   +

E11   From a Supine Position, with arms in High Position, palms up:
Sit up, raising legs to touch toes with hands on '1'. Return to starting position on '2'.

2   1

E12   From a Sitting Position, with arms in High Position:
Twist and lower trunk, rolling to left side to a basic prone position with arms overhead on '1 - 2'. Return to starting position on '3 - 4'. Repeat to right side.

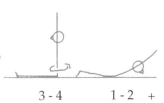

3 - 4   1 - 2   +

15 Back and Lower Trunk Strengthening Exercises

**E1   From a Prone Position, with arms in
Side Shoulder Position, palms
down:**
Raise arms, bending trunk backwards
on '1 - 2'. Return to starting position
on '3 - 4'.

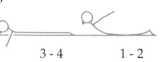

3 - 4   1 - 2

E2   From a Basic Kneeling Position:
Reach forwards to a supported position with arms extended in line with
trunk, pressing chest 3 times on '1 - 2
- 3'. Return to starting position on '4'.

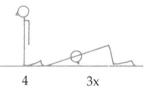

4   3x

**E3   From a Prone Position, with arms in
Side Shoulder Position, palms
down:** Raise arms and legs, bending
trunk backwards on '1 - 2'. Return to
starting position on '3 - 4'.

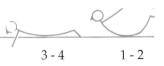

3 - 4   1 - 2

**E4   From a Prone Straddle Position,
with arms in Side Shoulder Position,
palms down:**
Clasping hands behind back, bend
trunk backwards 3 times on '1 - 2 - 3'.
Return to starting position on '4'.

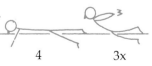

4   3x

**E5 From a Prone Position, with arms
in High Position and palms down:**
Raise arms, bending trunk backwards
on '1'. Return to starting position on
'2'. Raise legs on '3'. Return to starting position on '4'.

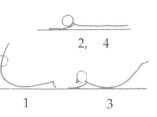

**E6 From a Prone Straddle Position,
with arms in Side Shoulder Position,
palms down:**
With trunk bending backwards and
legs raised, clap hands in high position
3 times on '1 - 2 - 3'. Return to starting position on '4'.

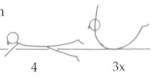

E7 From a Supported Prone Position:
Raise hips until arms are extended in
line with trunk, and press chest down
3 times on '1 - 2 - 3'. Return to starting position on '4'.

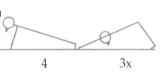

**E8 From a Prone Straddle Position,
with arms in deep position, palms
down:** With support from hands, bend
trunk backwards on '1 - 2'. Return to
starting position on '3 - 4'.

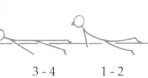

**E9 From a Prone Position, with arms in
High Position, palms down:**
Raise left arm and bend trunk backwards, exchanging arm positions in
slow and fast rhythms.

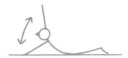

**E10 From a Prone Position, with arms in
High Position, palms down:**
Raise left leg, bending hips backwards, exchanging leg positions in
slow and fast rhythms.

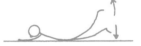

**E11 From a Prone Position, with arms in
High Position, palms down:**
Bend trunk backwards, and circle
arms in a counterclockwise direction
times on '1 - 2 - 3'. Return to starting
position on '4'.

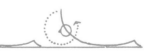

4   3x

**E12 From a Prone Position, with arms in
High Position, palms down:**
Raise arms and legs, bending trunk
backwards on '1'. Raise straddled legs
and swing arms sideways on '2'.
Close legs and return arms to high
position on '3'. Return to starting
position on '4'.

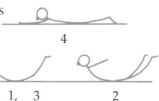

4

1,   3   2

Notes

Notes